Goji Berry

A Beginner's 3-Step Quick Start Guide to Incorporating Goji Berries for Health Benefits, With Sample Recipes

BRANDON GILTA

Disclaimer

By reading this disclaimer, you are accepting the terms of the disclaimer in full. If you disagree with this disclaimer, please do not read the guide.

All of the content within this guide is provided for informational and educational purposes only, and should not be accepted as independent medical or other professional advice. The author is not a doctor, physician, nurse, mental health provider, or registered nutritionist/dietician. Therefore, using and reading this guide does not establish any form of a physician-patient relationship.

Always consult with a physician or another qualified health provider with any issues or questions you might have regarding any sort of medical condition. Do not ever disregard any qualified professional medical advice or delay seeking that advice because of anything you have read in this guide. The information in this guide is not intended to be any sort of medical advice and should not be used in lieu of any medical advice by a licensed and qualified medical professional.

The information in this guide has been compiled from a variety of known sources. However, the author cannot attest to or guarantee the accuracy of each source and thus should not be held liable for any errors or omissions.

You acknowledge that the publisher of this guide will not be held liable for any loss or damage of any kind incurred as a result of this guide or the reliance on any information provided within this guide. You acknowledge and agree that you assume all risk and responsibility for any action you undertake in response to the information in this guide.

Using this guide does not guarantee any particular result (e.g., weight loss or a cure). By reading this guide, you acknowledge that there are no guarantees to any specific outcome or results you can expect.

All product names, diet plans, or names used in this guide are for identification purposes only and are the property of their respective owners. The use of these names does not imply endorsement. All other trademarks cited herein are the property of their respective owners.

Where applicable, this guide is not intended to be a substitute for the original work of this diet plan and is, at most, a supplement to the original work for this diet plan and never a direct substitute. This guide is a personal expression of the facts of that diet plan.

Where applicable, persons shown in the cover images are stock photography models and the publisher has obtained the rights to use the images through license agreements with third-party stock image companies.

Introduction

You might have noticed goji berries at the supermarket and been curious about what exactly they are.

Goji berries are a type of berry that is red and originate from a plant that is native to China. The plant that produces goji berries is known by its scientific name, Lycium barbarum. Goji berries have been utilized for their medicinal properties for hundreds of years in traditional Chinese medicine. It is possible to hear people refer to them as wolfberries.

Even though research on goji berries is still ongoing, there is some preliminary evidence that suggests these little red fruits may offer a variety of health benefits. These benefits include boosting the immune system, protecting against age-related eye damage, reducing inflammation, and containing antioxidants that may have positive effects on one's health.

There are a variety of grocery shops and online vendors that sell dried and fresh goji berries; if you are interested in incorporating them into your diet, you can locate them. You may also acquire them in the form of a powder or dietary supplement.

However, before beginning to take any dietary supplements, it is essential to have a conversation with your primary care physician about the possibility of interactions between the supplements and the prescriptions you are already taking.

In this beginner's guide, we'll deep dive into the following subtopics about goji berries:

- History of goji berry
- Goji berry nutritional facts
- Benefits of goji berry
- Use cases of goji berry
- Potential risks and side effects of goji berry
- Tips on buying goji berry
- A potential 3-step guide on how to incorporate goji berries into your life
- 11 goji berry recipes

Read on to learn more about goji berries and their potential health benefits.

Table of Contents

History of Goji Berry 1

Goji Berry Nutritional Facts 3

Benefits of Goji Berries 5

Use Cases of Goji Berries 8

Tips on Buying Goji Berries 16

A Potential 3-Step Guide on How to Incorporate Goji Berries Into Your Life 18

11 Goji Berry Recipes 21

HISTORY OF GOJI BERRY

As intriguing as the fruit itself is, the history of the goji berry is just as fascinating. This little berry is native to Asia and has been employed in the practice of traditional Chinese medicine for hundreds of years. However, only in recent times has the majority of the world become aware of the numerous health benefits that it offers.

Goji berries are believed to have originated in China, where they have been farmed for hundreds of years. The Chinese Emperor Shen Nung referred to the goji "Gou Qi" berry's therapeutic benefits in his book titled "Shen Nung Pen Ts'ao Ching" between the years 200 and 250 AD. This is the oldest known mention of the goji "Gou Qi" berry.

Since that time, the Goji berry has been utilized in traditional Chinese medicine to treat a wide range of conditions, including diabetes and hypertension, amongst others. As a result of the high quantities of vitamins, minerals, and antioxidants that it contains, the Goji berry has experienced a surge in popularity in recent years as a superfood in the Western world.

The consumption of goji berries is at an all-time high right now. It may be found in a wide variety of products, ranging from energy bars and supplements to smoothies and juices.

And as more and more people become aware of the numerous positive effects it has on their health, its popularity is expected to continue to rise.

GOJI BERRY NUTRITIONAL FACTS

Goji berries are a good source of vitamins A and C. They also contain iron and fiber. One ounce (28 grams) of dried goji berries contains about:

- Calories: 98
- Fat: 0.1 grams
- Carbs: 21.6 grams
- Fiber: 3.6 grams
- Protein: 4 grams
- Vitamin C: 15% of the Daily Value (DV)
- Vitamin A: 501% of the DV
- Iron: 11% of the DV

A study on the nutritional content of goji berries was carried out in 1988 by the Beijing Nutrition Research Institute to have a deeper understanding of the subject. According to the findings of the research, goji berries have a higher concentration of beta carotene than carrots, a higher concentration of iron than spinach, 500 times more vitamin C by weight than oranges, over 18 different amino acids, 21 different trace minerals, and significant amounts of vitamins B1, B2, B6, and E. The research also revealed that berries are an excellent source of carotenoids and contain essential fatty acids in their composition (more than any other known food).

Goji berries have an astonishingly high level of antioxidants in their natural content. An ORAC scale, also known as an Oxygen Radical Absorbance Capacity test, was developed by researchers working for the USDA at Tufts University in Boston. This test demonstrated that goji berries have ten times the antioxidant capacity of blueberries and five times the antioxidant capacity of prunes. These findings provided more evidence that goji berries deserve their status as a superfood.

BENEFITS OF GOJI BERRIES

Though more research is needed, there is some evidence to suggest that goji berries may offer certain health benefits. Here's a look at some key findings from recent studies:

Packed with antioxidants: According to several studies, the goji berry contains a high concentration of antioxidants. Antioxidants are known to assist in preventing cell damage and reducing inflammation. Polyphenols are a type of antioxidant that may be found in goji berries. These polyphenols are hypothesized to play a role in the prevention of both cancer and cardiovascular disease.

More vitamins and minerals: Traditional Chinese medicine has recognized the benefits of the goji berry for many decades, and with good cause. This little red fruit may be little, but it packs a significant nutritional punch thanks to its abundant vitamin and mineral content. Goji berries provide more than 500% of the Recommended Daily Intake (RDI) of vitamin C in just one serving, making them an ideal choice for those looking to get their vitamin C fix. In addition to this, they are an excellent source of fiber, iron, and calcium.

Anti-inflammatory: The Goji berry is a type of fruit that can only be found in China. For hundreds of years, it has been utilized in the traditional medical practices of China. There are a variety of medical applications for the plant's berries, leaves, and roots all of which may be found in nature. It is believed that the goji berry possesses anti-inflammatory effects, and as a result, it is occasionally used as a treatment for illnesses such as arthritis and joint pain.

Goji berries have also been demonstrated to be useful in lowering inflammation in the gut, which can contribute to improved gut health. This finding comes from a few different research. In addition to these benefits, the goji berry is known to strengthen the immune system and enhance circulation. Although further study is required to verify these advantages, the goji berry is a healthy and all-natural cure that has been utilized in traditional Chinese medicine for hundreds of years.

Improves blood circulation: Because of their beneficial effects on one's health, goji berries have been highly sought after for a long time. It is believed in traditional Chinese medicine that they can increase blood circulation and assist in the prevention of conditions such as anemia.

The findings of recent scientific research have shown that goji berries do have a beneficial impact on one's blood circulation. Consuming goji berries, which have been the subject of several studies, has been proven to contribute to an increase in the creation of red blood cells, which are responsible for transporting oxygen throughout the body.

In addition, goji berries include significant concentrations of iron, which is a mineral that is necessary for the body's cardiovascular system to operate effectively. As a consequence of this, consuming goji berries consistently can assist to guarantee that your blood is circulating effectively and that your cells are receiving the oxygen they require.

Adaptogens: Adaptogens are chemicals that assist the body in dealing with stress and maintaining a state of equilibrium. Goji berries are frequently referred to as adaptogens due to their beneficial effects on the body. It is believed that the use of goji berries in traditional Chinese medicine can assist in the treatment of both tiredness and anxiety.

Extract of goji berries has been proven in a few trials to be effective in lowering the levels of stress in rats. In human investigations, the extract of goji berries has also been proven to boost cognitive performance and reduce weariness. The first findings of a study on the benefits of goji berries on stress and exhaustion are encouraging; nonetheless, there is still a need for more investigation into this topic.

Goji berries are a real superfood that provides a wide variety of advantages to one's health. There is no question in anyone's mind that these small red fruits are beneficial to your health; nevertheless, further study is required to validate all of the possible health advantages of goji berries.

USE CASES OF GOJI BERRIES

The Goji berry is an exceptionally healthy fruit that is loaded with various vitamins, minerals, and free radical-fighting antioxidants. The term "superfood" is used to describe the goji berry rather frequently. Take a look at some of the following examples of how goji berries may be put to use:

Weight Loss: One of the most well-known advantages of consuming goji berries for your health is its capacity to facilitate weight loss. The goji berry is low in calories but high in fiber, which helps you feel full and satisfied after eating even though it has fewer calories than other berries.

In addition, goji berries have been shown to contain a substance known as lycopene, which has been demonstrated to speed up the metabolism and aid in the breakdown of fat. Goji berries are an excellent food choice to include in your diet if one of your goals is to reduce one's body fat percentage.

Eye protection: Goji berries are an excellent source of a wide variety of antioxidants, including carotenoid antioxidants like beta-carotene and zeaxanthin. These nutrients play a significant part in preventing the damage that can be induced by exposure to UV radiation in the eyes.

In addition, goji berries have been demonstrated to lessen the incidence of cataracts and other age-related visual issues. This is likely due to the high quantities of vitamin C that are found in goji berries. As a consequence of this, including goji berries in your diet regularly may help to safeguard your eyesight as you become older.

Boost immune system: Goji berries have been utilized for their medicinal properties for hundreds of years in traditional Chinese medicine. These tangy, ruby-colored berries are extremely beneficial to one's health due to the abundance of minerals and antioxidants that they contain. Goji berries provide a particularly significant boost to one's immune system. They have the potential to assist in the fight against infections and protect the body against pathogenic bacteria and viruses.

Additionally, goji berries assist in the enhancement of circulation and contribute to an increase in the creation of white blood cells. Because of this, consuming them is a wonderful approach to strengthening the immune system and maintaining overall bodily health.

Skin health: It is believed that the carotenoids and other nutrients found in goji berries, which may be found in the form of these little red fruits, are healthy for the skin. Carotenoids are potent antioxidants that can help to protect the skin from damage caused by free radicals. Carotenoids are found in a variety of fruits and vegetables.

Goji berries also include vitamins A and C, both of which are necessary ingredients in the manufacture of collagen.

Collagen is a kind of protein that aids in maintaining the elasticity and young appearance of the skin.

In addition, goji berries are an excellent source of fiber, which is known to facilitate the elimination of toxins from the body and the promotion of skin that is clear and radiant. Because of these benefits, including goji berries in your diet might potentially help enhance the health of your skin.

Heart Health: The goji berry has several wonderful health advantages, one of which is the excellent influence it has on the health of the heart. One of the compounds found in goji berries is called quercetin, and research has shown that it can decrease both blood pressure and cholesterol levels. In addition to its role as an antioxidant, quercetin has a role in preventing damage to the heart. If you want to enhance the health of your heart, including goji berries in your diet is an excellent method to accomplish this goal.

Protects against cancer: Goji berries have been demonstrated to help guard against cancer by lowering inflammation and stifling the growth of cancer cells, according to research conducted on the subject. Goji berries are an excellent source of antioxidants as well as polysaccharides, both of which are thought to strengthen the immune system and assist the body in its battle against the disease. As a consequence of this, consuming goji berries as part of your diet may assist in lowering the likelihood that you may acquire cancer.

Brain Health: Goji berry consumption has been shown to have beneficial benefits not just on the cardiovascular system but also on the brain. There is a component in goji berries called zeaxanthin, and research has shown that it can increase cognitive performance and protect the brain from the decrease that comes with aging.

Zeaxanthin is an antioxidant that has a role in assisting in the protection of the brain against damage brought on by free radicals. If you are seeking strategies to boost the health of your brain, including goji berries in your diet is an excellent approach to accomplish this goal.

Liver Protection: There is a correlation between maintaining a regular diet of goji berries and enhanced liver function. This can most likely be attributed to the goji berry's ability to shield the liver from the damaging effects of oxidative stress. A situation known as oxidative stress occurs when there is an excessive amount of a group of reactive oxygen species present in the body. This can cause harm to the cells and can result in inflammation. The Goji fruit has a significant amount of antioxidants, which work to eliminate the damaging effects of reactive oxygen species and shield cells from potential harm.

Hair growth: Goji berries are well known for their delightful flavor, but did you know that they also have potential benefits for your hair? These small red berries are loaded with minerals such as vitamin C, iron, and selenium, all of which are necessary for the formation of healthy hair. In addition, goji berries contain polysaccharides, which assist to stimulate hair follicles and encourage new hair development. This is an additional benefit of eating goji berries.

Kidney function: Traditional Chinese Medicine has made use of goji berries for hundreds of years due to the extensive array of health advantages that they offer, one of which is the enhancement of kidney function. Goji berries contain a wealth of antioxidants as well as other minerals that are beneficial to maintaining healthy kidney function.

For instance, they have a high concentration of vitamins C and A, both of which contribute to the kidneys' resistance to the damaging effects of oxidative stress. They also include important minerals such as iron, copper, and potassium, all of which are required for the kidneys to continue functioning normally and healthily. In addition, studies have indicated that the consumption of goji berries can increase blood circulation and decrease inflammation, both of which are helpful to the kidneys.

Regulates blood pressure: Goji berries have also been proven to assist in maintaining healthy blood pressure. This is because goji berries contain polysaccharides, which assist to relax the walls of blood vessels and lessen the pressure on the heart. As a result, the strain on the heart is reduced.

Additionally, goji berries have substances that assist to prevent platelets from sticking together, which helps prevent the formation of clots that can lead to strokes or heart attacks. This is an important benefit because both of these conditions can be fatal. Because of these factors, including goji berries in your diet may assist to maintain a healthy blood pressure range, which is beneficial to your overall health.

Regulates blood sugar: Goji berries have a high concentration of beneficial antioxidants and other chemicals that contribute to the regulation of blood sugar levels. Additionally, goji berries include both fiber and protein, both of which contribute to a reduction in the rate at which sugar is absorbed into the system. As a consequence of this, goji berries have the potential to be a useful instrument for controlling one's blood sugar levels.

Fertility: Increasing fertility is one of the many benefits attributed to the use of goji berries in Traditional Chinese Medicine. It is believed that the consumption of these berries can boost one's energy levels and general vitality, in addition to improving the quality of eggs and sperm. Goji berries have a high concentration of antioxidants, which shield eggs and sperm from the harmful effects of free radicals.

Additionally, it is believed that the berries might improve blood circulation, which makes them an invaluable tonic for couples who are trying to conceive a child. There is little question that for their size, goji berries pack a significant punch; nonetheless, further study is necessary before concluding that increased fertility may be achieved by the consumption of these berries. If a couple is having difficulty conceiving a child, adding goji berries to their diet may be an option that is worth exploring.

Stress Reduction: One of the most well-publicized advantages of goji berries is their capacity to alleviate stress. Researchers have shown that eating goji berries can help reduce levels of the stress hormone cortisol in the body. In addition, goji berries include significant concentrations of antioxidants, which are substances that can assist to defend the body against the potentially harmful effects of stress.

In addition, goji berries are an abundant source of several essential vitamins and minerals, such as vitamin C, iron, and selenium. These nutrients are needed for keeping a strong immune system, which can be compromised by prolonged stress and can be avoided by maintaining a healthy immune system. Therefore, including goji berries in your diet might help you minimize the amount of stress you experience and enhance your overall health.

Arthritis: It has also been found that the consumption of goji berries can be beneficial in the treatment of arthritis. This is due to the presence of molecules called carotenoids, which are known to protect joints from harm.

In addition, goji berries contain antioxidants that might aid in decreasing inflammation. Furthermore, goji berries are rich in vitamin C, which is needed for collagen formation. Proteins like collagen play an important role in maintaining the health and vitality of joints. As a result, including goji berries in your diet might help to alleviate some of the symptoms associated with arthritis.

As was just said, goji berries are associated with a diverse spectrum of positive health effects. If you are wanting to enhance your health, integrating goji berries into your diet is a fantastic place to start.

Potential Risks and Side Effects of Goji Berry

There are a few potential hazards and side effects that should be considered, even though goji berries are typically safe and well-tolerated by most people.

Goji berries have the potential to interact negatively with several drugs, including those used to treat diabetes, high blood pressure, and bleeding disorders. Therefore, before including goji berries in your diet, it is essential to discuss with your medical professional if you are already taking any kind of medicine.

Goji berries have been linked to several modest adverse effects, including gastrointestinal distress, bowel irregularity, and constipation. If you do suffer any of these unwanted effects, you must consume a diet high in fiber and water to mitigate their negative impact.

You may be allergic to goji berries if you have previously experienced allergic responses to other types of berries, such as strawberries or raspberries. Before taking goji berries, it is essential to get tested to see whether you have any food allergies.

Because there is little information on their safety, pregnant women and mothers who are still nursing should avoid eating goji berries.

These dangers are quite unlikely and, in the vast majority of instances, may be readily avoided according to the directions that have been provided. However, before ingesting goji berries, you must see your primary care physician. This is especially the case if you suffer from a medical condition or are using any kind of medicine.

TIPS ON BUYING GOJI BERRIES

If you are interested in including goji berries into your diet, there are a few things you should be aware of before purchasing them.

Goji berries can be purchased either dried, fresh, or ground into a powder. Goji berries, in their dried form, are the most popular type of berry that can be purchased, and they are stocked in virtually all health food stores. Fresh goji berries are harder to get by outside of Asia, but one can occasionally find them for sale in Asian grocery stores and specialty shops. Goji berry powder is also sold and may be acquired from a variety of different health food retailers.

It is essential to ensure that the goji berries you buy are of good quality before you spend your money on them. Goji berries should have a vibrant red color and be full-bodied. Steer clear of berries that have lost their vibrant color or have shrunken.

Checking the labels of goji berries to ensure that they are organic and free of pesticides is another vital step to take before purchasing them.

Consider buying goji berry powder if you're searching for an easy method to incorporate goji berries into your diet. This is a very popular option. Smoothies, yogurt, cereal, and even baked products can all benefit from the addition of goji berry powder.

A POTENTIAL 3-STEP GUIDE ON HOW TO INCORPORATE GOJI BERRIES INTO YOUR LIFE

Since you are now better informed about the goji berries and the positive effects they have on one's health, it is time to begin including them in your diet. This article will walk you through the process of doing so in three easy steps.

Step 1: Understand the difference between fresh and dried goji berries

The first thing you need to do is become familiar with the distinctions between fresh and dried goji berries. The dried form of goji berries is the more prevalent form and can be purchased at virtually any health food store. Fresh goji berries are harder to come by, but one can occasionally see them for sale at Asian stores.

Goji berries that have been dried have a chewy consistency and can be consumed as is or incorporated into other dishes. Fresh goji berries are more tender than their dried counterparts and can be consumed whole, blended into beverages, or incorporated into baked goods.

Step 2: Incorporate goji berries into your diet in a way that works for you

It's time to start incorporating goji berries into your life now that you have a better understanding of these superfoods and the possible advantages they offer. The next thing you need to do is figure out how best to include goji berries in your diet and stick to that routine. There are various methods to do this, but some suggestions include including dried goji berries into trail mix or yogurt, incorporating fresh goji berries into smoothies or baking dishes, or a combination of these two approaches.

Smoothies, yogurt, oats, or baked products are all excellent vehicles for the incorporation of goji berry powder. As goji berries can have a strong taste, it is important to begin using them in small amounts and gradually build up to the recommended serving size. And don't forget to pay attention to what your body is telling you; if you begin to notice any bad side effects, such as stomach trouble, it is better to cut back on the quantity you are ingesting or stop using the product entirely.

Step 3: Experiment with recipes that incorporate goji berries

It is time to start experimenting with different recipes that include goji berries now that you know where to obtain them and how to include them in your diet. There are several recipes for goji berry muffins, smoothies, energy bars, and other foods that may be found on the internet. And since they are so adaptable, the options for using goji berries are virtually limitless.

Therefore, use your imagination when you're cooking, and see what kinds of delectable recipes you can come up with. Who knows, maybe the dish you end up making is going to become your new go-to.

Goji Berry Breakfast Bowl

Start your day off right with this nutritious and delicious breakfast bowl! This bowl is packed with superfoods like goji berries, chia seeds, and acai powder. The goji berries add a sweet and tangy flavor, while the chia seeds provide a boost of fiber and protein.

Ingredients:

- 1/2 cup cooked quinoa
- 1/2 cup fresh blueberries
- 1/4 cup goji berries
- 1 tablespoon chia seeds
- 1 tablespoon acai powder

Instructions:

1. In a bowl, combine cooked quinoa, blueberries, goji berries, chia seeds, and acai powder.
2. Mix until everything is evenly combined.
3. Serve and enjoy!

Goji Berry Smoothie

This smoothie is the perfect way to get your daily dose of fruits and vegetables! The goji berries add a sweet and tangy flavor, while the spinach provides a boost of vitamins and minerals. The banana and almond milk make this smoothie creamy and delicious.

Ingredients:

- 1 banana
- 1 cup almond milk
- 1/2 cup goji berries
- 2 cups spinach

Instructions:

1. Add all of the ingredients to a blender and blend until smooth.
2. Pour into a glass and enjoy!

Goji Berry Salad

This salad is a great way to get your daily dose of fruits and vegetables! The goji berries add a sweet and tangy flavor, while the kale provides a boost of vitamins and minerals. The roasted almonds add a crunchy texture, while the balsamic vinegar adds a touch of acidity.

Ingredients:

- 1 cup kale, chopped

- 1/2 cup goji berries
- 1/4 cup roasted almonds
- 1 tablespoon balsamic vinegar

Instructions:

1. In a large bowl, combine the kale, goji berries, almonds, and balsamic vinegar.
2. Toss to combine.
3. Serve immediately.

Goji Berry Soup

This soup is a great way to get your daily dose of fruits and vegetables! The goji berries add a sweet and tangy flavor, while the carrots provide a boost of vitamins and minerals. The ginger gives this soup a spicy kick, while the coconut milk makes it creamy and delicious.

Ingredients:

- 1 tablespoon olive oil
- 1 onion, chopped
- 3 cloves garlic, minced
- 1 teaspoon fresh ginger, grated
- 4 cups vegetable broth
- 2 cups water
- 1 cup goji berries
- 1 large carrot, peeled and chopped
- 1 can of coconut milk
- salt and pepper to taste

Instructions:

1. Heat the olive oil in a large pot over medium heat. Add the onion, garlic, and ginger and cook until softened, about 5 minutes.
2. Add the vegetable broth and water and bring to a boil. Add the goji berries and carrot and cook until tender, about 10 minutes.
3. Puree the soup using an immersion blender or regular blender. Stir in the coconut milk and salt and pepper to taste. Serve hot.

Goji Berry Energy Bars

These energy bars are perfect for on-the-go snacking! They are packed with nutritious ingredients like goji berries, oats, flaxseed meals, and almond butter. These bars are also vegan and gluten-free, making them perfect for those with dietary restrictions.

Ingredients:

- 1 cup gluten-free oats
- 1/2 cup flaxseed meal
- 1/4 cup goji berries
- 1/4 cup almond butter
- 1/4 cup honey
- 1 tsp. vanilla extract

Instructions:

1. Preheat the oven to 350 degrees Fahrenheit. Line an 8x8-inch baking dish with parchment paper.
2. In a bowl, mix the gluten-free oats, flaxseed meal, goji berries, almond butter, honey, and vanilla extract until well combined.
3. Pour the mixture into the prepared baking dish and press it down firmly. Bake for 20 minutes or until golden brown. Allow cooling completely before cutting into bars.

Goji Berry Trail Mix

This trail mix is perfect for on-the-go snacking! It is packed with nutritious ingredients like goji berries, almonds, cashews, and dark chocolate chips. This mix is also vegan and gluten-free, making it perfect for those with dietary restrictions.

Ingredients:

- 1 cup goji berries
- 1 cup almonds
- 1 cup cashews
- 1/2 cup dark chocolate chips

Instructions:

1. In a large bowl, mix the goji berries, almonds, cashews, and dark chocolate chips.
2. Store in an airtight container for on-the-go snacking.

Goji Berry Pancakes

Start your day off right with these delicious pancakes! They are made with nutritious ingredients like goji berries, oat flour, flaxseed meal, and almond milk. These pancakes are also vegan and gluten-free, making them perfect for those with dietary restrictions.

Ingredients:

- 1 cup oat flour
- 1 tablespoon flaxseed meal
- 1 teaspoon baking powder
- A pinch of salt
- 1 cup almond milk
- 2 tablespoons maple syrup
- 1 teaspoon vanilla extract
- 1/4 cup goji berries, chopped

Instructions:

1. In a large bowl, whisk together the oat flour, flaxseed meal, baking powder, and salt. In a separate bowl, whisk together the almond milk, maple syrup, vanilla extract, and goji berries. Pour the wet ingredients into the dry ingredients and stir until well combined.
2. Preheat a griddle or frying pan over medium heat. Scoop 1/4 cup of batter onto the griddle or frying pan and cook for 2-3 minutes per side, or until golden brown. Serve with your favorite toppings!

Goji Berry Waffles

Start your day off right with these delicious waffles! They are made with nutritious ingredients like goji berries, oat flour, flaxseed meal, and almond milk. These waffles are also vegan and gluten-free, making them perfect for those with dietary restrictions.

Ingredients:

- 1 cup oat flour
- 1/4 cup flaxseed meal
- 1 teaspoon baking powder
- 1/4 teaspoon salt
- 1/2 cup almond milk
- 1/4 cup maple syrup
- 2 tablespoons olive oil or melted coconut oil
- 1 teaspoon vanilla extract
- 1/2 cup goji berries

Instructions:

1. Preheat your waffle iron. In a large bowl, whisk together the oat flour, flaxseed meal, baking powder, and salt.
2. In a separate bowl, whisk together the almond milk, maple syrup, olive oil or coconut oil, and vanilla extract.
3. Pour the wet ingredients into the dry ingredients and stir until well combined. Gently fold in the goji berries.

4. Pour about 1/2 cup of batter into your preheated waffle iron and cook for about 5-7 minutes, or until the waffle is golden brown and cooked through.
5. Repeat with the remaining batter.
6. Serve warm with your favorite toppings!

Goji Berry Muffin Bites

These muffin bites are perfect for on-the-go snacking! They are made with nutritious ingredients like goji berries, oat flour, flaxseed meal, and almond milk. These muffin bites are also vegan and gluten-free, making them perfect for those with dietary restrictions.

Ingredients:

- 1 cup oat flour
- 1/4 cup flaxseed meal
- 1 teaspoon baking powder
- 1/2 teaspoon salt
- 1 cup almond milk
- 1/4 cup maple syrup
- 2 tablespoons olive oil or melted coconut oil
- 1 teaspoon vanilla extract
- 1/2 cup goji berries, chopped

Instructions:

1. Preheat your oven to 350 degrees Fahrenheit. To make the oat flour, combine the oat flour, flaxseed

meal, baking powder, and salt in a large basin and mix together.

2. In a separate dish, combine the maple syrup, olive oil or coconut oil, vanilla extract, and almond milk by whisking all of the ingredients together.

3. After pouring the liquid components into the bowl containing the dry ingredients, give it a good swirl until everything is incorporated. The chopped goji berries should be incorporated carefully.

4. Put one level spoonful of the batter into each well of a small muffin tray. Bake the muffins for 12 to 15 minutes, or until they have a golden brown color all the way through and are completely cooked.

5. It should be let to cool for five minutes before being removed from the tin. Prepare and serve either hot or at room temperature.

Goji Berry Ice Cream

This ice cream is the perfect summer treat! It is made with nutritious ingredients like goji berries, almond milk, and cashew butter. This ice cream is also vegan and gluten-free, making it perfect for those with dietary restrictions.

Ingredients:

- 1 can of full-fat coconut milk
- 1/2 cup almond milk
- 1/2 cup maple syrup
- 1/2 cup cashew butter
- 1 teaspoon vanilla extract

- 1/4 cup goji berries, chopped

Instructions:

1. Put all of the ingredients into a powerful blender and process until the mixture is completely smooth. The liquid should be poured into an ice cream maker and frozen by the instructions provided by the manufacturer. You may either serve it right now or put it in the freezer for later.

Goji Berry Tart

This tart is the perfect special occasion treat! It is made with a nutritious goji berry filling and a gluten-free crust. This tart is also vegan, making it perfect for those with dietary restrictions.

Ingredients:

For the crust:

- 1 1/2 cups almond flour
- 1/4 cup tapioca flour
- 1/4 teaspoon salt
- 1/4 cup coconut oil, melted
- 1 tablespoon maple syrup

For the filling:

- 1 cup goji berries
- 1/2 cup almond milk

- 1/4 cup maple syrup
- 1 tablespoon tapioca flour

Instructions:

1. Preheat your oven to 350 degrees Fahrenheit. To prepare the crust, first put the almond flour, tapioca flour, and salt into a big basin and mix them. After the coconut oil and maple syrup have melted, pour them into the bowl and whisk until they are well incorporated.
2. Apply pressure to the dough and press it into a tart pan with a detachable bottom measuring 8 inches. While you are making the filling, put the crust in the freezer to keep it cold.
3. To prepare the filling, place all of the ingredients into a blender with a lot of power and process them until they are completely smooth. Pour the filling into the crust that has been made.
4. Bake the tart for 30 to 35 minutes, or until it has a golden brown color all the way through and is completely cooked. It should be allowed to cool for five minutes before being removed from the pan. Prepare and serve either hot or at room temperature.

Summary

Goji berries are believed to be a "superfood" owing to the high levels of antioxidants and nutrients that they contain. These berries have been utilized traditionally in Chinese medicine for hundreds of years. They are often offered for sale in dried form or as an ingredient in dietary supplements; however, certain markets also carry them in their fresh form. Goji berries are a nutritious complement to any diet since they have a somewhat low-calorie count, as well as because they do not contain any cholesterol or salt. In addition to this, they are an excellent source of fiber, vitamin C, iron, and a variety of other vital vitamins and minerals.

In addition, the chemicals included in goji berries have been shown to help protect against inflammation and the effects of aging. Consuming goji berries may assist improve blood sugar management, lower cholesterol levels, and promote improved heart health, according to the findings of several studies; nevertheless, there is still a need for more studies in this field. You may eat fresh, dried, or cooked goji berries, and they are also frequently used in beverages, cereals, trail mixes, baked products, and other types of mixes and dishes.

If you want to give goji berries a try, you should be sure to get them from a reliable retailer so you don't get a bad batch. In addition, you can get them in supplement form at a lot of different health food stores. However, before using any supplements, you must consult with your primary care physician or another healthcare expert.

When ingested in moderation, goji berries do not pose a health risk for the vast majority of people. However, if you are pregnant or nursing, you should limit your consumption of goji berries as much as possible since they may contain components that might be hazardous to your developing child if consumed in big quantities. Additionally, goji berries have the potential to interact with several different drugs; therefore, you must consult with your primary care physician before incorporating them into your diet if you are already taking any kind of medication daily.

Goji berries, in general, are a fruit that is packed with nutrients, can be consumed in a variety of different ways, and may offer some potential health advantages.

FAQ

1. What are goji berries?

Goji berries are a type of berry that is tiny and red. They are produced by a plant that is native to China. The plant that produces goji berries is known by its scientific name, Lycium barbarum. Goji berries are a type of fruit that has been used in traditional Chinese medicine for hundreds of years. These berries are said to provide a wide range of health advantages.

2. What do goji berries taste like?

The flavor of goji berries can be described as sweet with a hint of sourness. They are typically added to trail mix or granola, but they are also delicious when consumed on their own as a snack.

3. What are the health benefits of goji berries?

It is believed that eating goji berries can have a range of positive effects on one's health, including enhancing one's immune system, enhancing circulation, and providing protection against cardiovascular disease and cancer. Nevertheless, there is currently no proof from scientific research to back up these assertions.

4. Are there any side effects associated with consuming goji berries?

After taking goji berries, some people may have some moderate adverse effects, such as stomach trouble, diarrhea, or dizziness. These side effects are usually short-lived. If you start to feel any significant negative effects, you should immediately stop eating goji berries and contact a medical practitioner.

5. How many goji berries should I eat per day?

Due to the lack of scientific evidence to support any particular amount of goji berry consumption, there is no suggested daily intake of goji berries. On the other hand, daily use of goji berries in amounts up to 30 grams (approximately 1 ounce) is not thought to pose any health risks.

6. Can I grow my goji berry plant?

If you reside in a region that has a warm environment, then you have a good chance of successfully cultivating a goji berry plant in your own house. You may get goji berry plants for sale at some nurseries and on some websites that sell gardening supplies.

7. Where can I buy goji berries?

You may purchase goji berries at selected health food stores or from select internet sellers. They are frequently offered for sale in a dried or powdered form.

8. How should I store goji berries?

Dried goji berries have a shelf life of up to six months if they are kept in an airtight container in a dry and cold environment. If you have fresh goji, you should put them in the refrigerator as soon as possible and utilize them within two to three days.

References

7 Goji Berry Benefits Backed by Science. 7 Aug. 2018, https://www.medicalnewstoday.com/articles/322693.

"15 Benefits of Goji Berries, Nutrition, Side Effects, & Dosage." STYLECRAZE, 31 July 2013, https://www.stylecraze.com/articles/best-health-benefits-of-goji-berries/.

Chen, Jianjun, et al. Gojiberry Breeding: Current Status and Future Prospects. IntechOpen, 2018. www.intechopen.com, https://doi.org/10.5772/intechopen.76388.

Dube, Parul. "Goji Berry: Nutrition Facts, Benefits, and Side Effects." Blog - HealthifyMe, 10 Feb. 2022, https://www.healthifyme.com/blog/goji-berry/.

FoodData Central. https://fdc.nal.usda.gov/fdc-app.html#/food-details/173032/nutrients. Accessed 25 Nov. 2022.

Goji Berries: Ancient Remedy Finds New Popularity | Down to Earth Organic and Natural. https://www.downtoearth.org/articles/2009-03/32/goji-berries-ancient-remedy-finds-new-popularity. Accessed 25 Nov. 2022.

"Goji Berries: Nutrition, Benefits, and Side Effects." Healthline, 8 Sept. 2020, https://www.healthline.com/nutrition/goji-berry.

Ma, Zheng Feei, et al. "Goji Berries as a Potential Natural Antioxidant Medicine: An Insight into Their Molecular Mechanisms of Action." Oxidative Medicine and Cellular Longevity, vol. 2019, Jan. 2019, p. 2437397. PubMed Central, https://doi.org/10.1155/2019/2437397.

www.ingramcontent.com/pod-product-compliance
Lightning Source LLC
Chambersburg PA
CBHW051404150726

48000CB00003B/1326